Navigating the Dark Realities of Perimenopause

A Comprehensive Guide to the Hidden Struggles and Triumphs

Ruth M. Smith

Table of Contents

Chapter 1

UNDERSTANDING PERIMENOPAUSE

As a lady, If you're in your late 30s to early 40s, you wake up in a sweat at night, your periods are irregular and are occasionally accompanied by profuse bleeding (or scarcely any flow at all) — then chances are, you're going through perimenopause.

While your symptoms may seem erratic and beyond your control, it's vital not to panic or to feel overwhelmed by this often puzzling new phase.

Instead, the finest method to counteract your perimenopause is by understanding more about the change that is happening in your body, and why it happens. Once you understand the essentials, you'll be more equipped to handle this transitional time, head-on.

What is the perimenopause?

Perimenopause is the transitional stage preceding menopause — that is, the natural end of menstruation and your ability to reproduce. Peri is Greek meaning "around" or "near", and it is at this lead-up stage that women begin to notice symptoms of the oncoming menopause, from restlessness and night sweats to vaginal dryness. Although it may vary, perimenopause lasts for about 8-10 years, with most women entering it around the age of 39-49.

Is "perimenopause" the same as "premenopause"?

Although you could hear these expressions being used interchangeably, they mean two completely different things. The North American Menopause Society (NAMS) describes perimenopause as "perimenopause is the transition phase into menopause that typically lasts for about six years", whereas premenopause is "the time between a woman's first period and the onset of perimenopause" — essentially, her reproductive years.

What causes the perimenopause?

But, what's going inside the body to cause this change? Well, it's all down to the level of oestrogen in your body which begins to surge and decrease inconsistently during the perimenopause. As such, many women will begin to notice that their monthly periods become unpredictable in duration and flow — with excessive bleeding, or almost any flowing at all. Let's take a look at the role of oestrogen during perimenopause in a little more detail below.

PERIMENOPAUSE AND OESTROGEN

Many of the changes you'll experience throughout the perimenopause are related to oestrogen — or a lack thereof.

The amount of oestrogen in our body rises and falls within a set level throughout the menstrual cycle during our peak reproductive years. Since oestrogen levels are largely controlled by two hormones, follicle-stimulating hormone (FSH) and luteinizing (LH).

FSH stimulates the follicles — the fluid-filled sacs in the ovaries that contain the eggs — to generate oestrogen. Once the quantity of oestrogen hits a specified threshold, the pituitary gland is prompted by the brain to cut off the FSH and create a surge of LH.

It is this surge of LH that prompts the ovary to release the egg from its follicle (ovulation). After ovulation the remaining follicle releases progesterone and oestrogen in preparation for pregnancy, which in turn causes the levels of FSH and LH to decline. In the occurrence of ovulation that does not result in pregnancy, progesterone drops, menstruation takes place and the cycle begins again.

As your ovaries age though, they release less and fewer hormones, meaning that there is less FSH and LH to regulate oestrogen production. This leads a woman's oestrogen levels to fluctuate during perimenopause, finally switching off totally once the menopause arrives.

Other factors include:
Perimenopause generally begins in a woman's late 30s to early 40s, but it can start earlier or later for some individuals. This phase can extend anywhere from a few months to several years and is distinguished by numerous hormonal, physiological, and psychological changes.

Understanding the causes and mechanisms causing perimenopause demands digging into the complexities of female reproductive biology.

Hormonal Changes:

Perimenopause is primarily caused by changes in hormonal production and regulation, particularly involving the hormones oestrogen and progesterone. Throughout a woman's reproductive years, the ovaries generate these hormones in cyclical patterns that govern the menstrual cycle and influence many parts of a woman's physiology.

As a woman reaches perimenopause, her ovaries begin to generate less oestrogen and progesterone, resulting in irregular menstrual episodes and a range of symptoms.

Follicular Decline:

A significant feature contributing to perimenopause is the continuous reduction in the amount and quality of ovarian follicles. Ovarian follicles are tiny sacs within the ovaries that store growing eggs. With ageing, the ovaries have fewer viable follicles, leading to decreased egg production and uncertain ovulation. This reduction in follicle quality could contribute to variations in hormone levels and cycle irregularities.

Fluctuating Hormone Levels:
The hormonal fluctuations during perimenopause could be fairly unpredictable. Oestrogen levels can rise and decrease in irregular ways, contributing to symptoms like hot flashes, nocturnal sweats, mood swings, and fluctuations in menstrual flow. Progesterone levels may also become unpredictable, leading to changes in mood, sleep issues, and other symptoms.

Impact of Reproductive Aging:
As a woman matures, her body's response to reproductive hormones becomes less efficient. The communication between the

ovaries, pituitary gland, and hypothalamus (known as the hypothalamic-pituitary-ovarian axis) gets blocked, leading to irregular ovulation and menstruation.

Genetic Factors:
Genetics have a key in determining the age at which perimenopause begins. If a woman's mother or elder sisters experienced early perimenopause, she might likewise be more prone to make the shift at an earlier age.

Lifestyle and Environmental Factors:
Certain lifestyle and environmental factors can influence the timing and degree of perimenopause symptoms. Smoking, for example, has been connected with early onset of menopause.

Additionally, a high-stress lifestyle, poor food, lack of physical activity, and obesity might lead to hormone imbalances and worsen perimenopausal symptoms.

Medical Conditions and Treatments:
Certain medical illnesses and medical interventions can change the timing and progression of perimenopause. Conditions such as polycystic ovarian syndrome (PCOS) or thyroid difficulties could alter hormone levels and menstrual regularity.

Medical interventions like chemotherapy or some medicines can potentially trigger early menopause or worsen perimenopausal symptoms.

<u>Symptoms of the perimenopause</u>

Now that you know what is occurring to your body hormonally, we address the symptoms that could develop as a result of fluctuating oestrogen levels. Some of the key identifiers are:

Perimenopause is a transitional phase in a woman's life that precedes menopause. During this phase, the body undergoes enormous hormonal changes, leading to a variety of physical, emotional, and cognitive issues.

The symptoms of perimenopause could vary greatly in strength and length from woman to woman. It's vital to recognize and understand these symptoms to effectively manage and navigate this transitional phase. Here is a full review of the symptoms of perimenopause:

1. Irregular Menstrual Cycles:
- One of the defining symptoms of perimenopause is irregular menstrual cycles.
- Menstrual flow may become heavier or lighter, and the length between periods may fluctuate.
- Some cycles could be longer or shorter than average, and skipping periods or

having two periods in one month is not uncommon.

2. Hot Flashes and Night Sweats:

- Hot flashes are abrupt sensations of high heat that can induce flushing, perspiration, and a rapid heartbeat.
- Night sweats are hot flashes that occur during sleep, generally leading to disrupted sleep patterns.

3. Mood Changes:

- Hormonal fluctuations during perimenopause might lead to mood swings, irritability, and heightened sensitivity to stimuli.
- Some women may endure concern or feelings of melancholy, and there is an elevated chance of developing severe depression at this time.

4. Sleep Disturbances:

- Hormonal variations could contribute to difficulties going to sleep or staying asleep, contributing to insomnia.
- Night sweats can also affect sleep patterns, resulting in tiredness and daytime sleepiness.

5. Vaginal Changes:

- Decreased oestrogen levels can contribute to vaginal dryness, discomfort, and soreness, making sexual intercourse less pleasant.
- Some women may report an increased sensitivity to vaginal infections.

6. Changes in Sexual Desire:

- Hormonal alterations can modify libido and sexual desire, resulting in changes in sexual satisfaction and closeness.

7. Urinary Symptoms:

- Some women may develop urine incontinence, increased urinary urgency, or more frequent urinary tract infections.
- These symptoms are often related with the weakening of pelvic muscles and tissues owing to hormonal changes.

8. Cognitive Changes:

- Some women describe having "brain fog," memory lapses, and trouble concentrating during perimenopause.
- While the particular relationship between hormone changes and cognitive performance is still being researched, these modifications are not unusual.

9. Weight Changes and Metabolism:

- Hormonal imbalances could contribute to weight gain, especially in the abdomen area.
- Changes in metabolism can make it more tough to maintain or lose weight during perimenopause.

10. Skin and Hair Changes:

- Decreased oestrogen levels can lead to changes in skin elasticity, adding to dryness and wrinkles.
- Hair may grow thinner and more fragile.

11. Bone Health:

- Oestrogen has a key role in maintaining bone density, hence decreasing levels during perimenopause can elevate the risk of osteoporosis.

12. Cardiovascular Changes:

- Oestrogen exerts preventative actions on the cardiovascular system. As oestrogen levels fall, there can be an increased risk of heart disease.

13. Headaches:

- Some women may experience an increase in the frequency or severity of headaches during perimenopause.

14. Joint and Muscle Pain:

- Hormonal fluctuations might lead to joint and muscular discomfort, analogous to symptoms reported during premenstrual syndrome (PMS).

15. Changes in Breasts:

- Breasts could become more sensitive or lumpy, which can sometimes be misunderstood as an indicator of breast cancer. Regular breast self-examinations are necessary.

16. Digestive Issues:

- Some women may have digestive difficulties such as bloating, indigestion, and changes in bowel patterns.

17. Changes in Cholesterol Levels:

- Hormonal changes can modify cholesterol metabolism, leading to alterations in lipid levels in the blood.

18. Allergies and Skin Sensitivities:

- Some women can have an increase in allergies or heightened skin sensitivities during perimenopause.

19. Gum and Dental Changes:

- Hormonal variations might influence oral health, resulting in alterations in gum health, higher susceptibility to gum disease, and probable dry mouth.

20. Changes in Vision:

- Some women may notice changes in eyesight, including dry eyes and trouble concentrating on close objects.

21. Hair Growth Changes:

- While hair on the head could get thinner, some women might report more facial hair growth or hair formation in unusual spots due to hormonal imbalances.

22. Tinnitus and Ear Issues:

- Hormonal changes might contribute to changes in ear pressure, leading to sensations of ringing in the ears (tinnitus) or variations in hearing.

23. Electric Shock Sensations:

- Some women experience sudden, fleeting electric shock symptoms, known as "brain zaps," during perimenopause.

24. Changes in Body Odour:

- Hormonal fluctuations can contribute to changes in body odour, with some women detecting modifications in their natural scent.

25. Food Cravings and Aversions:

- Hormonal changes could alter food preferences, resulting in new cravings or aversions to particular meals.

26. Tingling Sensations:

- Some women may have tingling or numbness in their extremities, often attributed to hormonal changes altering nerve function.

27. Gastrointestinal Symptoms:

- Hormonal imbalances can disrupt the gastrointestinal system, resulting in symptoms such as bloating, gas, and changes in bowel patterns.

28. Electric Sensations in the Skin:

- Some women could report sensations of tingling, burning, or electric shocks in the skin, often referred to as "paresthesias."

29. Changes in Body Temperature Regulation:

- Fluctuations in oestrogen levels can compromise the body's ability to regulate temperature, leading to sensitivity to cold or heat.

30. Anxiety and Panic Attacks:
- Hormonal changes could contribute to feelings of worry and panic attacks, especially in women who are vulnerable to anxiety problems.

31. Breathing Changes:
- Some women may have alterations in respiratory patterns, sometimes leading to shortness of breath or a feeling of air hunger.

32. Dizziness and Lightheadedness:
- Hormonal variations could alter blood pressure and fluid balance, resulting in occasional dizziness or sensations of lightheadedness.

33. Sensitivity to Light and Sound:
- Some women could report heightened sensitivity to light and sound during perimenopause.

34. Muscle Tension and Pain:

- Hormonal changes can add to muscle tension and pain, particularly in the back and neck.

35. Increased Body Hair Shedding:

- While some women experience increased facial or body hair growth, others may observe higher shedding of hair from the scalp.

36. Changes in Nail Health:

- Hormonal alterations can lead to changes in the strength and health of nails.

37. Metallic Taste in the Mouth:

- Some women report experiencing a metallic taste in their tongue, which can be due to hormonal changes.

38. Changes in Body Composition:

- Hormonal swings can contribute to changes in fat distribution, with some women noticing increased belly fat.

39. Heightened Sensitivity to Pain:
- Some women could endure higher sensitivity to pain or changes in pain tolerance during perimenopause.

40. Changes in Body Fluids:
- Hormonal alterations can modify the content of physiological fluids, perhaps resulting in changes in saliva, tears, and vaginal secretions.

PERIMENOPAUSE VS MENOPAUSE

While both stages influence a woman's reproductive system, and have many of the same symptoms, there are some variances between the two stages. For example, women will experience their periods for the first part of the perimenopause, which means they may still be able to get pregnant.

While at the menopause stage, your ovaries stop releasing eggs and produce most of their oestrogen required for reproduction. Ultimately, it's good to think of perimenopause as the build-up to the major event of menopause.

How do I know I am perimenopausal?

If you are experiencing any of the symptoms listed above, it could be worth arranging an appointment with your GP to make the diagnosis of perimenopause. Before you do, it's worth reading our guide on perimenopause symptoms for a more in-depth review.

What are the four stages of Perimenopause?

According to Canadian endocrinologist Professor Jerilynn Prior, perimenopause can unfold across four stages.

- Very early perimenopause, when periods are still regular.
- Early menopausal transition, from the onset of irregular cycles.
- Late menopause transition, from the first cycle of more than 60 days.
- Late perimenopause, which is 12 months from your final period.

Does perimenopause affect fertility?

During perimenopause, levels of these hormones rise and fall sporadically, causing irregular periods, reduced ovulation, and some of the symptoms associated with menopause—such as fluctuating moods and night sweats. 1 As such, the ups and downs of these reproductive hormone levels make it difficult to become pregnant

Do you ovulate during perimenopause?

During perimenopause, blood levels of these hormones can both recede and potentially surge. This leads not just to irregular periods but also to unpredictable ovulation cycles. Throughout this time, the ovaries are continuing to release eggs.

Chapter 2

<u>DEBUNKING COMMON MISCONCEPTIONS</u>

Perimenopause, commonly referred to as the "menopausal transition," is a challenging phase in a woman's life that comes with various hormonal changes and symptoms. However, despite its relevance, there are several typical misconceptions and misunderstandings concerning perimenopause that can lead to confusion and needless anxiety.

Addressing these misunderstandings is crucial for offering accurate information and better-supporting women as they handle this natural transition. Here are some of the most popular myths around perimenopause:

1. Perimenopause and Menopause Are the Same:

<u>Misconception:</u> Many persons use the phrases "perimenopause" and "menopause" interchangeably, assuming they refer to the same phase.

<u>Clarification:</u> Perimenopause is the transitional phase leading up to menopause, which is the moment when a woman has not had a menstrual cycle for 12 consecutive months. Menopause marks the end of reproductive capacity, while perimenopause spans the years preceding it.

2. Perimenopause Only Affects Older Women:

<u>Misconception:</u> It's often considered that perimenopause only develops in a woman's late 40s or early 50s.

<u>Clarification:</u> Perimenopause can start as early as a woman's late 30s or even earlier for some women. Age of onset varies due to inherited factors, health history, and lifestyle choices.

3. Hormonal Changes Are the Same for Everyone:

<u>Misconception:</u> It's widely thought that all women suffer the same hormonal changes and symptoms during perimenopause.

<u>Clarification:</u> Hormonal changes are individualised. While oestrogen levels decline, the patterns and intensities of symptoms could differ greatly. Some women could experience significant symptoms, while others might have a very straightforward transition.

4. Perimenopause Is Just About Hot Flashes:

<u>Misconception:</u> Hot flashes are frequently highlighted as the major symptom of perimenopause.

<u>Clarification:</u> While hot flashes are a well-known symptom, perimenopause involves a wide range of physical, emotional, and cognitive changes, including irregular periods, mood swings, sleep issues, vaginal changes, and more.

5. Hormone Therapy Is the Only Solution:

Misconception: Hormone therapy (HT) is generally thought of as the only approach to control perimenopausal symptoms.

Clarification: While HT can be successful for some women, it's not the lone choice. Lifestyle modifications, non-hormonal drugs, and holistic treatments can help relieve symptoms. Treatment selections should be tailored to each woman's particular needs and preferences.

6. You Can't Get Pregnant During Perimenopause:

Misconception: Many women feel that pregnancy is not attainable during perimenopause.

Clarification: As ovulation becomes less predictable but doesn't totally cease, it's still possible to become pregnant during perimenopause. Birth control methods of contraception are indicated if pregnancy is not desired.

7. Perimenopause Is Just a Physical Phase:

Misconception: Perimenopause is generally seen only as a physiologic phase without emotional or psychological impact.

Clarification: Hormonal changes might impact mood, cognitive function, and emotional well-being. Anxiety, depression, and mood swings are frequent emotional symptoms during perimenopause.

8. Symptoms Are Permanent:

Misconception: Some women fear that perimenopausal symptoms would continue indefinitely.

Clarification: While symptoms can remain, they often improve during menopause as hormonal oscillations settle. However, some symptoms include vaginal changes and bone density concerns could require continuous care.

9. Perimenopause Is a Disease:

Misconception: Perimenopause is sometimes incorrectly considered as an illness or health condition.

Clarification: Perimenopause is a natural and normal phase of a woman's life, not a sickness. It's a biological process that signifies the change from reproductive to non-reproductive years.

10. All Symptoms Require Medical Treatment:

Misconception: Some women feel that all perimenopausal symptoms necessitate medical care.

Clarification: While medical treatment can help reduce symptoms, some women might find relief through lifestyle modifications, self-care approaches, and non-prescription therapies.

11. Perimenopause Happens Suddenly:

<u>Misconception:</u> Many people assume that perimenopause happens fast and without notice.

<u>Clarification:</u> Perimenopause is a gradual process that occurs over several years. The start of symptoms and changes could vary, and some women might not even identify they're in perimenopause until they experience more pronounced symptoms.

12. You Have No Control Over Symptoms:

<u>Misconception:</u> Some women feel that they have little control over perimenopausal symptoms and must tolerate them.

<u>Clarification:</u> While hormonal changes are a natural feature of perimenopause, lifestyle factors such as nutrition, exercise, stress management, and sleep can greatly impact the degree and frequency of symptoms.

13. Perimenopause Is the Same for Every Culture:

<u>Misconception:</u> The experience of perimenopause is sometimes assumed uniform across all cultures.

<u>Clarification:</u> Cultural and cultural elements can influence how women experience and view perimenopause. Attitudes toward ageing, openness about discussing menopause, and available support networks can differ.

14. Emotional Changes Are Just a "Midlife Crisis":

<u>Misconception:</u> Emotional changes during perimenopause are often seen as a mere midlife crisis.

<u>Clarification:</u> Emotional fluctuations are real and can be linked to hormone imbalances. They may include mood swings, anxiety, and depression, which should be acknowledged and addressed as part of the perimenopausal experience.

15. Perimenopause Is Over Once Menopause Begins:

Misconception: People assume that once menopause starts, the symptoms of perimenopause vanish.

Clarification: While certain symptoms may improve following menopause, some may continue for a period. Additionally, new challenges connected to postmenopausal health can emerge.

16. Hormone Therapy Is Always Risky:

Misconception: Hormone therapy is typically regarded as dangerous and risky for all women.

Clarification: Hormone therapy can be safe and successful when administered appropriately and under the counsel of a healthcare practitioner. The decision to seek hormone treatment should be based on an individual's medical history and risk factors.

17. Natural Remedies Are Infallible:
Misconception: Some feel that all-natural remedies are always safe and beneficial in managing perimenopausal symptoms.
Clarification: While natural therapies can be beneficial for some women, they might not work for everyone. Consultation with a healthcare provider is needed to assure safety and efficacy.

18. Perimenopause Only Affects Physical Health:
Misconception: Perimenopausal symptoms are typically considered primarily physical, ignoring their impact on mental and emotional health.
Clarification: Perimenopause can lead to emotional and psychological changes, changing mood, cognitive function, and overall well-being.

19. You Can't Prepare for Perimenopause:

Misconception: Many women feel that there's no way to prepare for the rigours of perimenopause.

Clarification: Educating oneself about perimenopause, seeking support from healthcare professionals, and adopting healthy lifestyle practices can help women proactively manage and cope with symptoms.

20. Perimenopause Is a Sign of Aging Failure:

Misconception: Some women relate perimenopause with a sense of failure or loss due to ageing.

Clarification: Perimenopause is a natural and usual phase of life. Viewing it as a positive transformation and focusing on embracing personal growth and well-being might help modify this mentality.

Dispelling these fallacies about perimenopause is crucial for creating a solid understanding and healthy attitudes concerning this significant life phase.

When women are armed with right information and support, they can approach perimenopause with confidence, make informed decisions, and prioritise their well-being during the transition and beyond.

Chapter 3

<u>EXPLORING THE EMOTIONAL ANGUISH OF PERIMENOPAUSE</u>

When you think about perimenopause—the years preceding menopause—you may think of the physical symptoms: hot flashes, nocturnal sweats, and the ultimate loss of periods. But many people also experience mood difficulties at this period.

Mental health changes can have several causes. The hormone changes that impact your periods during perimenopause might affect your emotions too. Also, physical menopausal symptoms can lead to stress and tiredness, raising emotions.

On top of that, your 40s and 50s are a time when life's pressures can be highest. Many people in this age bracket are managing hard professions, raising younger children or sending older children off to college, and caring for ageing parents. All of this stress could add to mental health difficulties.

Mood fluctuations might feel like PMS. About 4 in 10 women have mood symptoms during perimenopause that are similar to PMS, or premenstrual syndrome. You can feel irritated, have poor energy, feel emotional and irritable, or have a hard time concentrating.

Unlike PMS, these symptoms may arise at periods unrelated to your menstrual cycle. Symptoms may occur for years with no pattern. This sort of mood fluctuation is known as perimenopausal mood instability.

Depression is frequent during perimenopause. Most researchers believe that the risk of depression increases during the menopause transition. Symptoms of depression include crying a lot, feeling hopeless or worthless, feeling numb, and losing interest in your regular activities.

You may experience nervousness also. There is limited data about anxiety during perimenopause, however, some women experience symptoms of anxiety at this time. Anxiety involves constant concern that gets in the way of your day-to-day life. You may experience muscle tightness, sweat, or nausea. Both depression and anxiety can make it hard to concentrate, sleep, and take care of yourself.

Research has indicated that around 23 percent of women will suffer mood swings throughout menopause. When we talk about menopausal mood swings, we're often talking to the mood fluctuations that occur throughout perimenopause. During this time, women may suffer substantial mood swings and may feel anxiety and depression for the first time in their lives.

The emotional variations experienced at this time can be considerable. They seem to come out of the blue and may be substantially more severe than anything encountered in the past. Many of my perimenopausal clients express that they feel out of control or as if they're "going mad."

It might be tough to maintain doing the activities they've always done when they find themselves exhausted, emotional, and even forgetful at times. Changes throughout this time of life affect nearly every part of a woman's life, with some finding mood swings the toughest thing to manage.

So, what causes perimenopausal mood swings?

Oestrogen reduction. Oestrogen—the major female sex hormone that is necessary for sexual development and for regulating a woman's menstrual cycle and reproductive system—is produced in the ovaries. Oestrogen has a dramatic impact on mood, largely by modifying levels of serotonin in the body.

Serotonin is a mood-balancing chemical that is sometimes called the "happiness hormone." During perimenopause, as oestrogen levels start to drop, so do our levels of serotonin. This is one of the reasons why we may feel more depressed and are more likely to cry at the drop of a hat than we would have been in the past.

Progesterone decline. The other main sex hormone in a woman's body is progesterone. Similarly to oestrogen, levels of progesterone begin to drop during perimenopause. As progesterone levels fall, oestrogen may become the dominant hormone, leading to irritability and depression.

Progesterone is responsible for calming the brain and promoting sleep; a reduction in progesterone can have the opposite effect. Low levels of progesterone are associated with a range of symptoms including sleep disturbances, migraines, hot flashes, and unexplained anxiety. The combination of these symptoms can have a major impact on mood.

Hormonal fluctuations. Hormones are complicated creatures, as are the human mind and body. Oestrogen doesn't just steadily drop. Instead, the production of oestrogen becomes unstable and unpredictable.

During the process of overall decrease, the ovaries may start to overcompensate in producing oestrogen, resulting in a hormonal surge. At other times, there will be a marked drop in oestrogen and these fluctuating levels may be particularly noticeable in the second half of a woman's cycle, following ovulation. These fluctuations can have a very destabilising impact on your moods.

Hormonal imbalance. When we're thinking about the impact of hormones on mood, we can't isolate one hormone at a time. Instead, we need to think about how these hormones work in combination with each other.

During perimenopause, the delicate balance of hormones is affected by the reductions and fluctuations mentioned above. For instance, when progesterone decreases, women can end up being "oestrogen dominant" which can cause a range of physical symptoms—such as bloating, decreased libido, and fatigue—as well as mental symptoms, including anxiety and depression.

Sleep disruptions. We all know the influence that poor sleep has on our mood (just think about how irritated and even easily agitated you were the last time you slept badly!). Many women experience severe sleep disturbances during perimenopause, even if they have never had difficulty sleeping before.

Changes in oestrogen and progesterone affect the function of other hormones that are essential for regulating bodily temperature. Hot flashes which are experienced at night—called night sweats—can adversely impact women's sleep patterns, with some women reporting waking up soaked in perspiration.

The hormonal swings noted above, which can create anxiety, mean that it can be difficult for women to fall asleep and can mean that they are sometimes quite abruptly woken up in an anxious or panicky condition.

Hot flashes. Sudden surges of heat, sometimes accompanied by uncontrollable sweating, are known as hot flashes. A normal hot flash will last between 30 seconds and 10 minutes.

Sometimes, they can be highly obvious to others, as the face reddens and many women feel embarrassed and nervous about experiencing a flash, which can stop them in their tracks. The difficulties in dealing with hot flashes can induce anxiety and depression in some people.

Other menopausal symptoms. Menopause is accompanied with a full array of symptoms, some of which women find quite unpleasant to live with.

These symptoms can include weight gain, diminished libido, vaginal dryness, sensitive breasts, excessive bloating, loss of breast fullness, thinning hair, and dry skin—in addition to hot flashes, sleeplessness, and hormonal mood swings!

Coping with a changing body, a changing sexual relationship, and everything else that is going on during perimenopause may be quite difficult and can have a huge affect on mood.

Pressured time of life. For many women, this midpoint in life also coincides with a high degree of pressure. The "sandwich generation" refers to people who are responsible for caring for children and their parents. Even if you don't have kids, you may find yourself faced with responsibilities for caring for older parents, holding down a job, and dealing with a myriad of other pressures.

Difficult transitions. Whether or not you have ever wanted children, or have had all the children you ever desired, menopause brings into sharp focus that your childbearing years are coming to an end.

This can be a difficult realisation for some women and perhaps more so for women who have experienced fertility issues in their lives or have "unfinished business" with regard to having children, perhaps because they never had a relationship in which they wanted to bring a child into the world. In those cases where women have had children, the "empty nest" can cause great distress and anxiety.

I've had several clients—including women whose focus was certainly not exclusively directed towards childrearing and the home—who have felt far more upset than they expected as their children leave home. Any life transition can be hard, and this is a transition that goes to the core identity and may involve a significant change in day-to-day life.

Existential terror. Many women face ageing with a sense of dread which is heightened by the fact that we live in a culture that prizes youth. Both women and men can face a sense of fear at this stage in their lives.

There's something about realising that, realistically, you're midway through your life. It makes you sit up and take stock. Some people might look over what they've done so far and feel a sense of regret. Some might take this as an opportunity to reassess what's working and what isn't. Some might feel overwhelmed at the thought of ageing and of having failed to achieve what they might have desired in their youth.

Menopausal mood swings can be severe, but it is important that there are very real physical changes that are happening in your body that are impacting how you feel and behave. If you are finding it hard to cope on your own, therapeutic approaches including CBT and hypnotherapy have a proven track record in helping manage symptoms and provide a complementary, or alternative, approach to conventional, bio-medical menopausal treatments.

The Emotional Turmoil of Perimenopause

Perimenopause, the transitional time leading up to menopause, is a significant and delicate stage in a woman's life. While the physical changes are often explored, the mental upheaval that often accompanies this phase is also important to explore.

The emotional roller coaster experienced during perimenopause can be severe, confusing, and tough to manage, impacting not only the woman going through it but also those around her.

Perimenopause typically begins several years before menopause, when a woman's ovaries start producing less oestrogen and progesterone. These hormonal fluctuations can trigger a range of physical and emotional symptoms, leading to what's often referred to as a "hormonal storm." The emotional turmoil of perimenopause arises from the intricate interplay between these hormonal changes, psychological factors, and life circumstances.

Emotional Symptoms of Perimenopause

1. <u>Mood Swings:</u> One of the most common emotional symptoms is mood swings. These rapid shifts in mood can go from euphoria to irritability, from calmness to intense frustration, sometimes within a matter of moments. The fluctuations in hormone levels, particularly oestrogen, can affect neurotransmitters that regulate mood, leading to these unpredictable emotional changes.

2. <u>Anxiety and Depression:</u> Many women experience heightened levels of anxiety and depression during perimenopause. Hormonal imbalances can influence brain

chemistry and exacerbate preexisting mood disorders or trigger new ones. Women who have a history of depression or anxiety might find that these conditions become more pronounced during this phase.

3. <u>Irritability and Anger:</u> Feelings of irritability and anger can be intense and overwhelming. Women might find themselves getting agitated more easily, reacting strongly to situations that wouldn't have bothered them before. These emotional responses can strain relationships and create a sense of isolation.

4. <u>Cognitive Changes:</u> Cognitive capacities like memory and focus could be reduced during perimenopause. "Brain fog," forgetfulness, and difficulty with multitasking are not atypical. These cognitive changes might contribute to emotions of discontent and decreased self-esteem.

5. <u>Exhaustion and Sleep disruptions:</u> Sleep disruptions and exhaustion are frequent physical symptoms of perimenopause, but they can also have a substantial impact on emotional well-being. Chronic sleep deprivation can lead to mood swings, anger, and an overall sense of emotional instability.

6. <u>Loss and Grief:</u> For some women, perimenopause can inspire feelings of loss and grief. The knowledge that fertility is decreasing, along with the change into a new era of life, can lead to a sense of mourning for one's youth and reproductive potential.

The Dynamics of Relationship Strains

<u>Communication Challenges:</u> Hormonal fluctuations during perimenopause can contribute to mood swings, impatience, and emotional sensitivity. These changes can make communication more complex, as

what might have been a minor issue could generate heightened emotional responses.

<u>Intimacy Concerns:</u> Vaginal dryness and changes in libido can impair sexual intimacy. Women might feel less comfortable or engaged in sexual engagement, leading to misunderstandings or feelings of rejection in their partners.

<u>Emotional Roller Coaster:</u> Mood swings, anxiety, and depression are prevalent during perimenopause. Partners and loved ones could find it difficult to negotiate these emotional fluctuations, leading to misunderstandings and tensions.

<u>Coping Differences:</u> Individuals have varied coping techniques for dealing with stress and emotional issues. While some might prefer isolation and self-reflection, others might crave more social connection. These differences can lead to misunderstandings and feelings of neglect.

<u>Changing Priorities:</u> Perimenopause is frequently a period of introspection and reevaluation of life goals and priorities. This shift in focus can lead to changes in daily routines, hobbies, and social interactions that might damage relationships.

Hormonal Changes and Sexual Impact

<u>Libido Fluctuations:</u> Hormonal shifts, particularly a drop in oestrogen levels, can lead to changes in sexual desire or libido. Some women could feel a decrease in sexual desire, while others might observe an increase owing to hormonal fluctuations.

<u>Vaginal Dryness:</u> Declining oestrogen levels can contribute to vaginal dryness, thinning of the vaginal walls, and less natural lubrication. This can result in discomfort, pain, or even bleeding during sexual intercourse.

Sensitivity Changes: Changes in hormone levels can lead to changed genital sensitivity, influencing the way women feel sexual stimulation. This can affect the time it takes to become aroused and the intensity of orgasms.

Mood and Arousal: Emotional fluctuations, including mood swings and anxiety, can alter sexual arousal and enjoyment. Stress and emotional issues might limit sexual responsiveness.

Professional and Societal Challenges of Perimenopause

Professional Challenges:

1. Productivity effect: The physical and emotional symptoms of perimenopause, such as weariness, mood swings, and cognitive changes, might affect a woman's productivity at work. Reduced focus, memory lapses, and decreased energy levels might affect job performance.

2. <u>Stigma and Silence:</u> Perimenopause is still a topic that is often stigmatised or ignored in professional contexts. Women might hesitate to disclose their experiences owing to fears of being viewed as unable or unstable.

3. <u>Workplace Support:</u> Many companies lack complete policies to support women experiencing perimenopause. Access to flexible work hours, breaks, or accommodations to manage symptoms can be limited.

4. <u>Misdiagnosis:</u> Some symptoms of perimenopause, such as anxiety and cognitive problems, could be mistaken as other disorders including stress or early-onset dementia. This can lead to ineffective therapies and more challenges.

5. <u>Age Discrimination:</u> Perimenopause frequently occurs throughout the late 40s to

early 50s, a time when women could also suffer age-related discrimination or biases in the job.

Societal Challenges:

1. <u>Taboo and Ignorance:</u> Societal taboos and a lack of information about perimenopause lead to a culture of silence. Many women feel unsupported and lonely owing to the lack of open communication.

2. <u>Expectations of Youthfulness:</u> Societal expectations of youthfulness can lead to women feeling compelled to hide their age-related problems. This pressure might hamper their ability to seek help or openly share their challenges.

3. <u>Media Representation:</u> The media typically presents women as permanently youthful and carefree, neglecting the realities of ageing and hormonal changes. This can generate unreasonable expectations and promote prejudices.

4. <u>Medical Disparities:</u> Medical research and therapies have historically focused more on men's health, resulting in a lack of full understanding of women's experiences during perimenopause.

Chapter 4

<u>**MEDICAL OPTIONS FOR PERIMENOPAUSE**</u>

Perimenopause, the transitional phase leading up to menopause, is characterised by hormonal imbalances that can result in a wide range of physical and mental problems. For women enduring distressing symptoms that significantly influence their quality of life, medical alternatives offer a pathway to symptom control and relief.

From hormone therapy to pharmaceutical and alternative treatments, comprehending the available medical alternatives is crucial for making educated decisions regarding one's health throughout this phase.

1. Hormone Therapy (HT):

Hormone treatment entails taking medications that contain hormones, commonly oestrogen or a combination of oestrogen and progesterone, to decrease perimenopausal symptoms. It's one of the most efficient techniques to alleviate symptoms linked with hormone swings.

- <u>Oestrogen Therapy:</u> Used largely for women who have had a hysterectomy (removal of the uterus), oestrogen therapy can help manage hot flashes, vaginal dryness, and mood swings.

- <u>Oestrogen-Progestin Therapy:</u> This combined therapy is intended for women who still retain their uterus. It can lower the danger of uterine cancer related to oestrogen therapy alone. It's effective for treating hot flashes, mood difficulties, and other symptoms.

2. Non-Hormonal Medications:
Some women prefer non-hormonal alternatives for several reasons, including

health difficulties or personal preferences. Non-hormonal medications can be effective in managing specific perimenopausal symptoms:

- <u>Selective Serotonin Reuptake Inhibitors (SSRIs) and Serotonin-Norepinephrine Reuptake Inhibitors (SNRIs):</u> These antidepressants are often used to manage mood changes, anxiety, and depression associated with perimenopause.

- <u>Gabapentin and Pregabalin:</u> These medications, normally used to treat nerve pain, can help alleviate hot flashes and mood issues.

- <u>Clonidine:</u> Originally a blood pressure medicine, clonidine can be used to treat hot flashes and nocturnal sweats.

3. Alternative Treatments:

Alternative remedies can offer comfort for women who prefer non-medication procedures or want to complement their treatment plan:

- <u>Herbal Supplements:</u> Some women obtain relief from symptoms utilising herbal supplements like black cohosh, red clover, or evening primrose oil. However, the effectiveness of these supplements varies and should be reviewed by a healthcare expert.

- <u>Mind-Body Therapies:</u> Techniques like yoga, tai chi, meditation, and deep breathing techniques can help regulate stress, anxiety, and mood swings.

- <u>Acupuncture:</u> Some women report fewer hot flashes and increased sleep following acupuncture sessions.

4. Individualised Approach:

Every woman's experience of perimenopause is unique. Factors such as medical history, overall health, and individual symptoms have a role in determining the most appropriate pharmacological solutions. Consulting with a healthcare specialist is crucial to determine the best approach for managing symptoms.

5. Risks and Benefits:

When contemplating medical treatments, it's crucial to assess the potential risks and benefits. Hormone therapy, for instance, carries hazards such as an increased risk of blood clots, stroke, and some malignancies. Non-hormonal drugs and alternative treatments also come with potential adverse effects and interactions.

6. Regular Follow-up:

Regardless of the chosen medical approach, frequent follow-up with a healthcare professional is important. Monitoring the efficacy of the therapy and altering the plan if necessary ensures that symptoms are addressed optimally.

7. Lifestyle Modifications:

In addition to pharmacological alternatives, lifestyle improvements can play a crucial role in treating perimenopausal symptoms. These adjustments can complement medical therapies and add to general well-being:

- <u>Healthy Diet:</u> A balanced diet rich in whole grains, fruits, vegetables, and lean proteins can give important nutrients to preserve hormonal balance and general health.

- <u>Regular Exercise:</u> Engaging in regular physical activity can help calm mood changes, enhance sleep quality, and reduce the risk of osteoporosis.

- <u>Stress Reduction:</u> Practising stress reduction tactics such as meditation, mindfulness, and deep breathing can help reduce anxiety and mood swings, and boost general emotional well-being.

- <u>Adequate Sleep:</u> Prioritising quality sleep by having a consistent sleep schedule, providing a comfortable sleep environment, and practising relaxing techniques helps reduce sleep troubles.

- <u>Limiting Caffeine and Alcohol:</u> Reducing caffeine and alcohol intake, especially in the evening, can lead to better sleep quality and minimise hot flashes.

8. Customised Approach:

Perimenopause is a time of transformation that affects each woman distinctively. What works well for one individual might not be suitable for another. Healthcare providers take into account aspects such as medical history, current health state, and personal preferences to build a tailored treatment plan.

9. Regular Check-ins:

Treatment options should involve regular check-ins with healthcare providers. Monitoring the success of the selected treatment and addressing any concerns or changes in symptoms ensures that women receive the assistance they need throughout the perimenopausal journey.

10. Empowerment and Education:

Understanding the available medical alternatives encourages women to take an active role in their perimenopausal health. Armed with knowledge about various treatments, risks, and advantages, women can engage in educated discussions with their healthcare providers to make decisions that accord with their objectives and preferences.

Medical solutions for perimenopause give a spectrum of possibilities to help women properly manage the varied range of symptoms that can emerge during this transitional phase. From hormone therapy to non-hormonal drugs, alternative treatments, and lifestyle modifications, the path to symptom relief is diverse and suited to individual needs.

By working closely with healthcare experts and making informed decisions, women can traverse perimenopause with a full strategy that enhances their well-being, quality of life, and overall health.

Chapter 5

EMPOWERING SELF-CARE STRATEGIES FOR NAVIGATING PERIMENOPAUSE

Perimenopause, the transitional phase leading up to menopause, is a time of profound physical, mental, and psychological changes. As women travel this altering road, practising self-care becomes crucial to preserving general well-being and enjoying this new chapter of life.

By practising appropriate self-care routines, women can withstand the difficulties of perimenopause with patience, grace, and a restored sense of empowerment.

1. Prioritise Sleep:

Quality sleep is crucial for reducing perimenopausal symptoms. Create a tranquil evening routine, follow a consistent sleep schedule, and create a comfortable sleep environment. Avoid coffee and screen time before bed to aid deep sleep.

2. Nourish Your Body:

A balanced diet rich in nutrients helps promote hormone balance and general well-being. Prioritise whole foods such as fruits, vegetables, whole grains, lean meats, and healthy fats. Stay hydrated and consider adding meals high in calcium and vitamin D to assist bone health.

3. Regular Physical Activity:

Engaging in regular exercise delivers various benefits during perimenopause. Physical activity can help calm mood changes, reduce stress, boost sleep quality, and preserve bone health. Aim for a combination of aerobic, strength training, and flexibility workouts.

4. Stress Management:

Practice stress-reduction practices such as meditation, deep breathing, yoga, and mindfulness. These tactics can help minimise anxiety, and mood fluctuations, and promote emotional well-being.

5. Stay Hydrated:

Drink plenty of water throughout the day to stay hydrated. Adequate hydration enhances skin health, cognitive function, and general energy.

6. Mind-Body Practices:

Engage in mind-body disciplines such as meditation, tai chi, or progressive muscle relaxation. These exercises can help reduce stress, boost relaxation, and enhance emotional resilience.

7. Seek Social Support:

Connect with friends, family, or support groups. Sharing experiences, concerns, and pleasures with others helps establish a sense of belonging and minimise feelings of loneliness.

8. Express Yourself:
Explore creative paths such as writing, art, music, or dancing. Expressing yourself creatively can act as a strong tool for processing emotions and fostering self-discovery.

9. Limit Caffeine and Alcohol:
Moderate your intake of caffeine and alcohol, especially at night. These chemicals might affect sleep habits and lead to mood fluctuations.

10. Educate Yourself:
Knowledge is empowering. Educate yourself about perimenopause to better understand the physical and emotional changes you're experiencing. This awareness can help you navigate this period with greater confidence.

11. Practice Self-Compassion:

Be nice and sympathetic to yourself. Embrace self-acceptance and understand that the hardships of perimenopause are a natural part of life's journey.

12. Set Boundaries:

Learn to set appropriate boundaries in multiple facets of your life, including job, relationships, and personal duties. Prioritise your well-being and make time for self-care without feeling guilty.

13. Pamper Yourself:

Indulge in self-care habits such as taking relaxing baths, obtaining massages, or indulging in activities that provide you joy and relaxation.

14. Maintain Regular Health Check-ups:

Regularly contact your healthcare practitioner for check-ups and screenings.

Discuss your perimenopausal symptoms and any worries you might have.

15. Listen to Your Body:
Pay heed to your body's signs and respond accordingly. Rest when you need to, and respect your body's need for self-care.

16. Practice Gratitude:
Cultivate a sense of appreciation by concentrating on the positive things of your life. Keeping a thanksgiving book or even taking a moment each day to reflect on what you're thankful for could boost your general attitude and mental well-being.

17. Learn to Say No:
Learning to say no when you're feeling overwhelmed or when a commitment doesn't connect with your well-being is a key self-care skill. Prioritise activities and duties that resonate with you.

18. Connect with Nature:

Spending time in nature may have a relaxing and refreshing effect. Take walks in green spaces, enjoy outdoor pastimes, and reconnect with the natural world to enhance your mood and reduce stress.

19. Plan for "Me Time":

Set out concentrated time for yourself each day. Whether it's reading, following a hobby, or simply relaxing, this time encourages you to refuel and focus on your own needs.

20. Explore Mindfulness:

Mindfulness includes being present in the moment without judgement. Engaging in mindfulness activities, such as mindful breathing or body scans, can reduce stress and promote emotional well-being.

21. Laugh and Have Fun:

Engage in things that bring joy and laughter into your life. Whether it's watching a comical movie, spending time with loved ones, or trying something new, laughter may be a strong stress relief.

22. Embrace Alone Time:
Alone time may be rejuvenating, allowing you to reflect, relax, and connect with yourself. Use this time to indulge in things you enjoy and enhance self-awareness.

23. Maintain a Supportive Routine:
Establish a daily routine that supports your physical and emotional well-being. This regimen can include exercise, good food, soothing activities, and proper sleep.

24. Celebrate Achievements:
Acknowledge and celebrate your achievements, no matter how modest. This action can enhance your self-esteem and reaffirm your sense of significance.

25. Positive Affirmations:

Use positive affirmations to fight negative self-talk and increase self-confidence. Remind yourself of your talents and potential.

26. Set Realistic Goals:

Set acceptable goals that fit with your priorities and energy levels. This can minimise emotions of overwhelm and create a sense of success.

27. Practise Deep Breathing:

Deep breathing exercises can boost the body's relaxation response, decreasing tension and providing a sensation of tranquillity.

28. Stay Curious:

Embrace a curious and open perspective. perspective difficulties with a readiness to learn and grow, fostering resilience and adaptability.

29. Embrace Change:

Perimenopause is a phase of transition. Embrace the changes as chances for growth and self-discovery rather than rejecting them.

30. Reflect and Adapt:
Regularly assess your self-care habits and make modifications as needed. Your demands may fluctuate over time, so remain varied in your approach.

Self-care during perimenopause encompasses an array of techniques that promote your physical, emotional, and psychological well-being. By adopting these self-care practices into your everyday life, you may handle the obstacles of perimenopause with grace, resilience, and a strong sense of self-empowerment.

Remember that taking care of oneself is not selfish; it's an essential investment in your overall health and quality of life. Embrace the journey of self-discovery and growth

that perimenopause brings, and emphasise
self-care as a crucial guiding light on your
route.